SOUTH BEACH

DIET COOKBOOK

Quick and simple recipes for beginners to loss weight with pictures | 21-day meal plan |

Keri Johnson

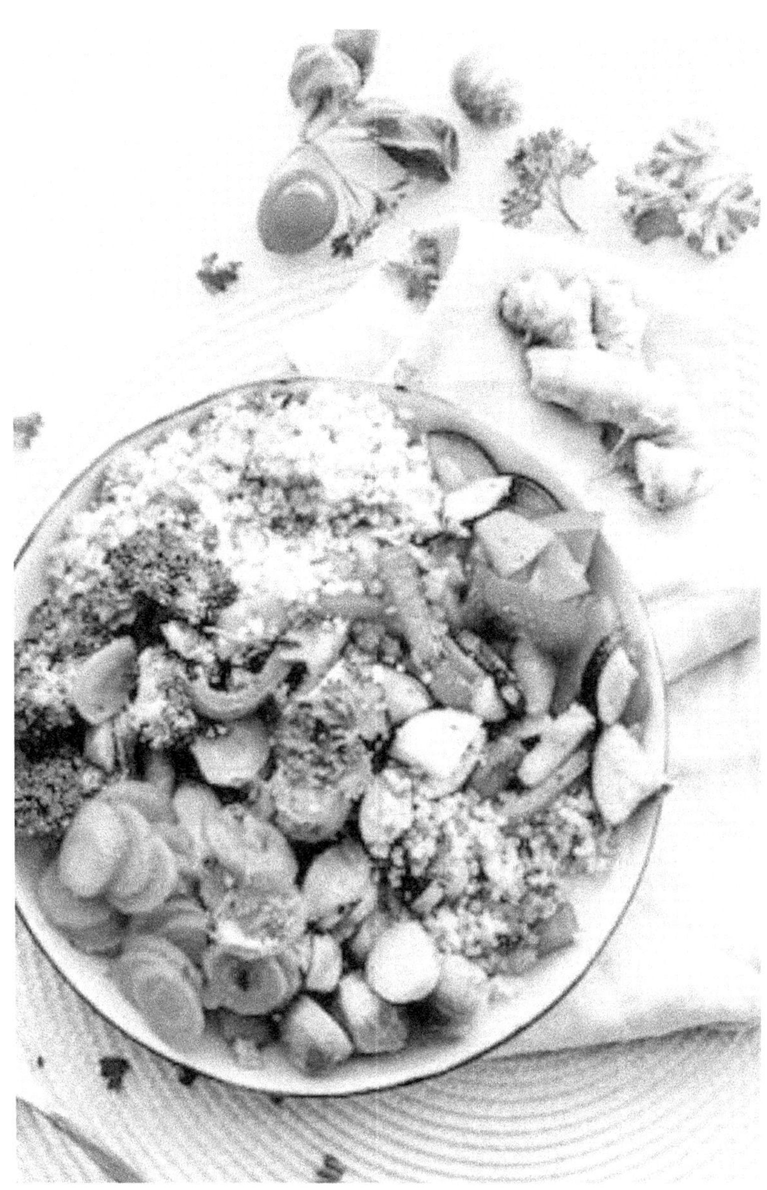

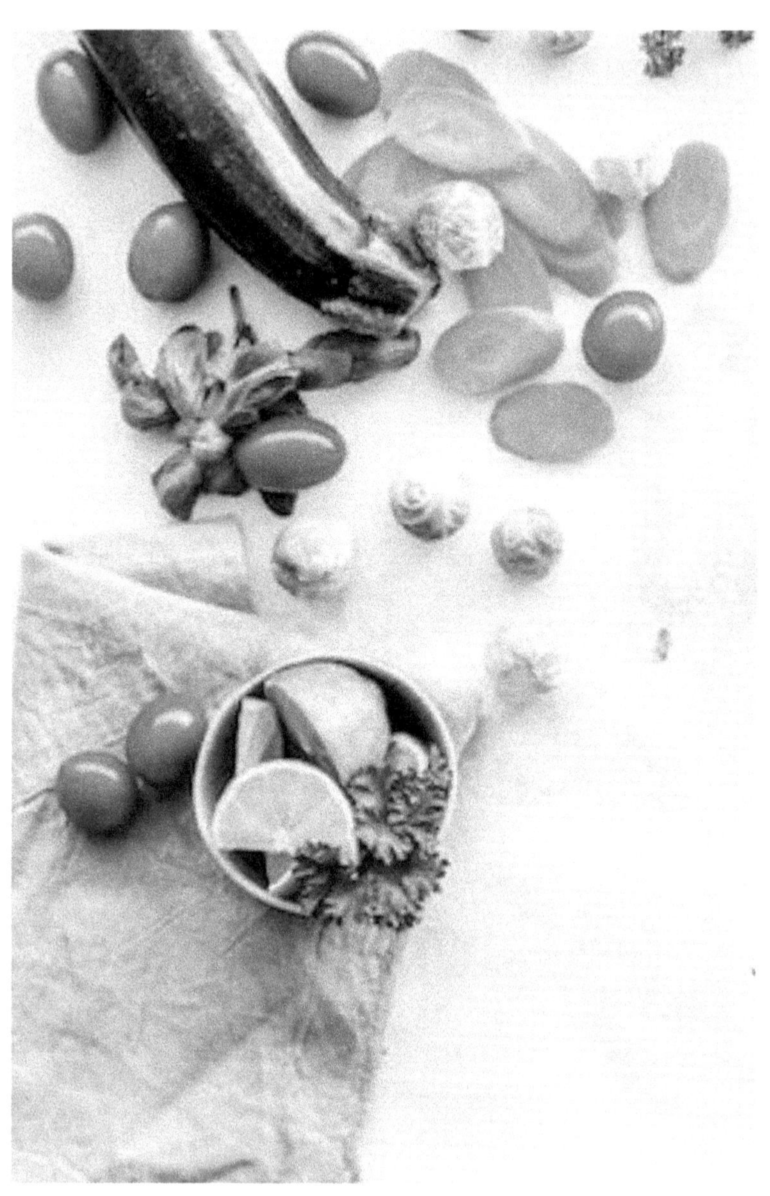

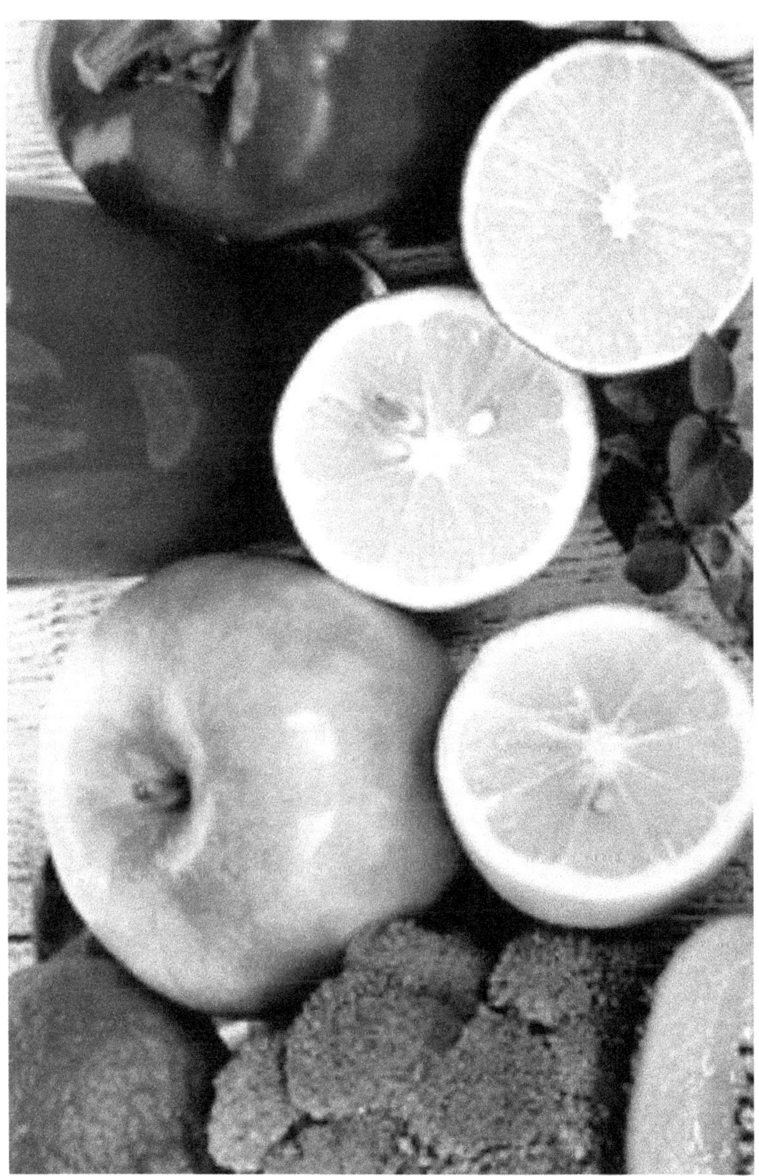

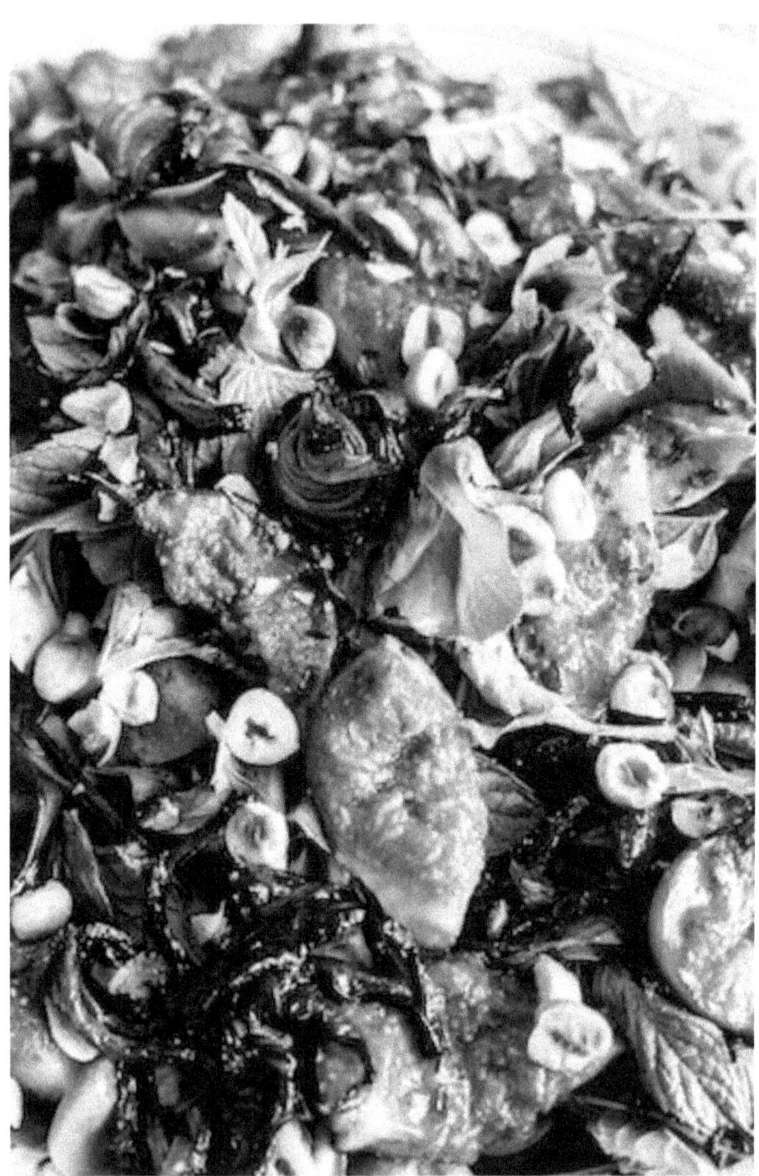

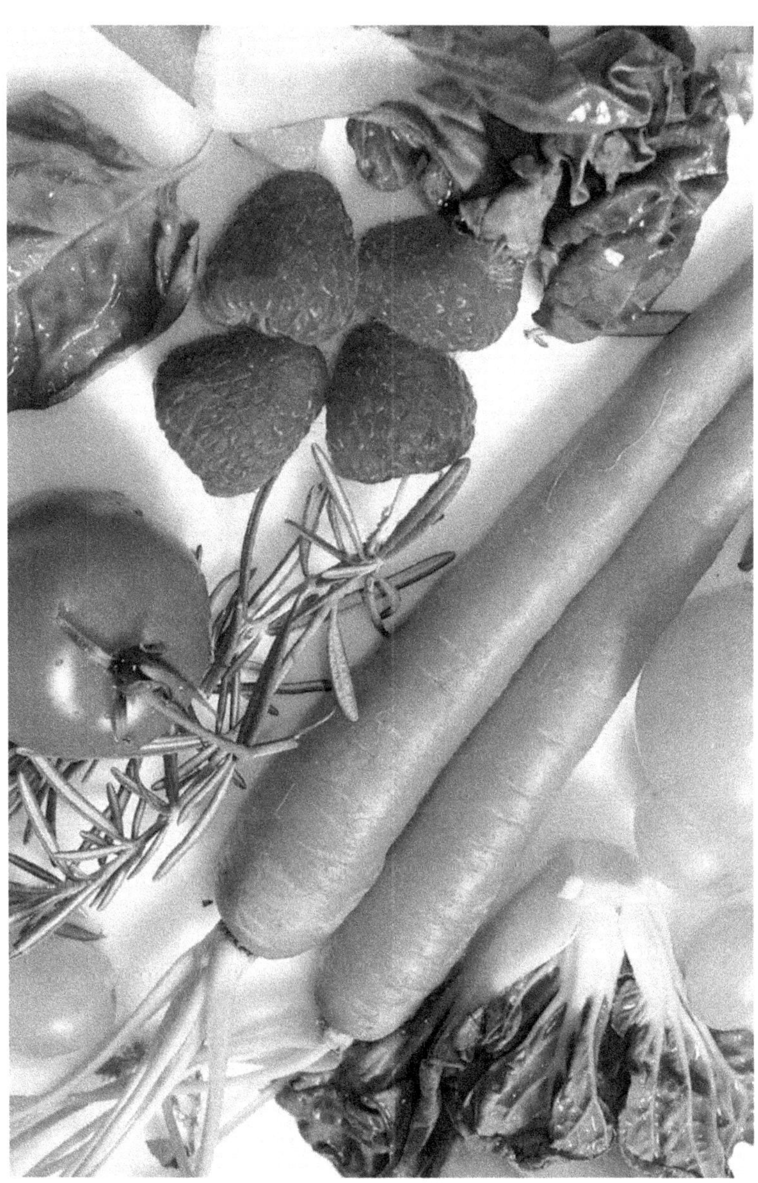

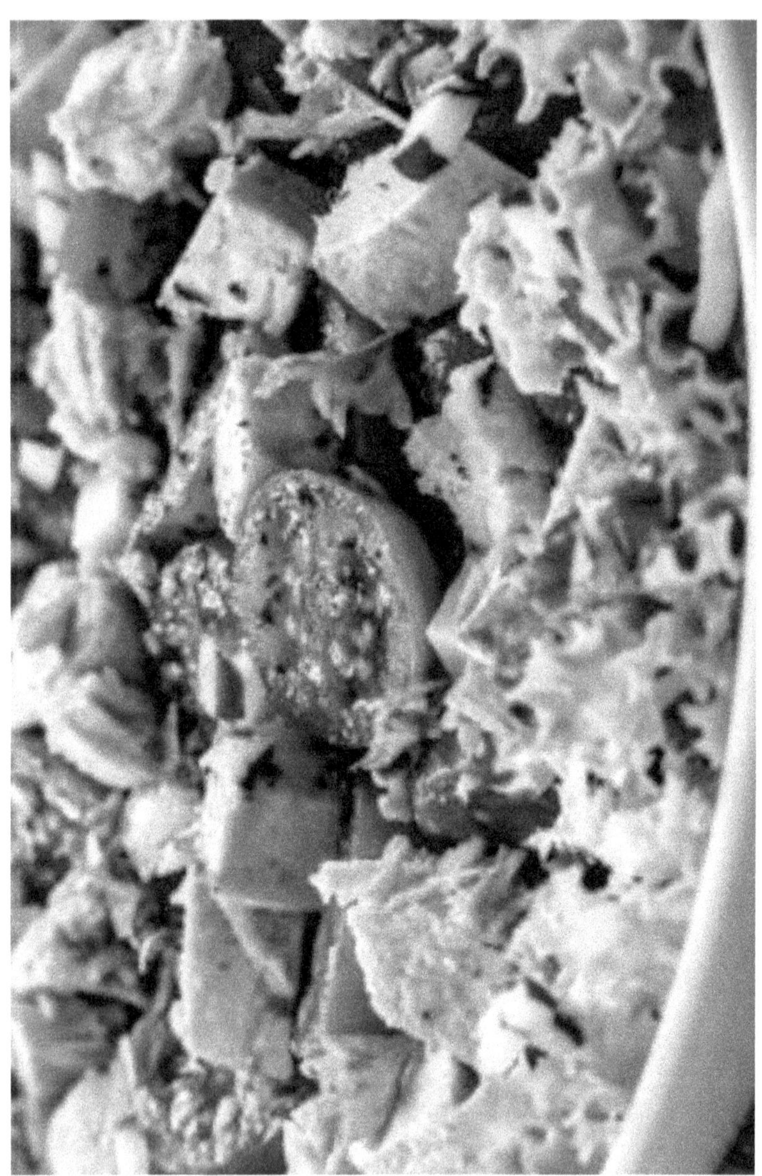

TABLE OF CONTENTS

CHAPTER FIVE   59

CHAPTER SIX   73

CHAPTER SEVEN   85

VEGETABLES AND FRUITS RECIPES FOR SOUTH BEACH DIET   85

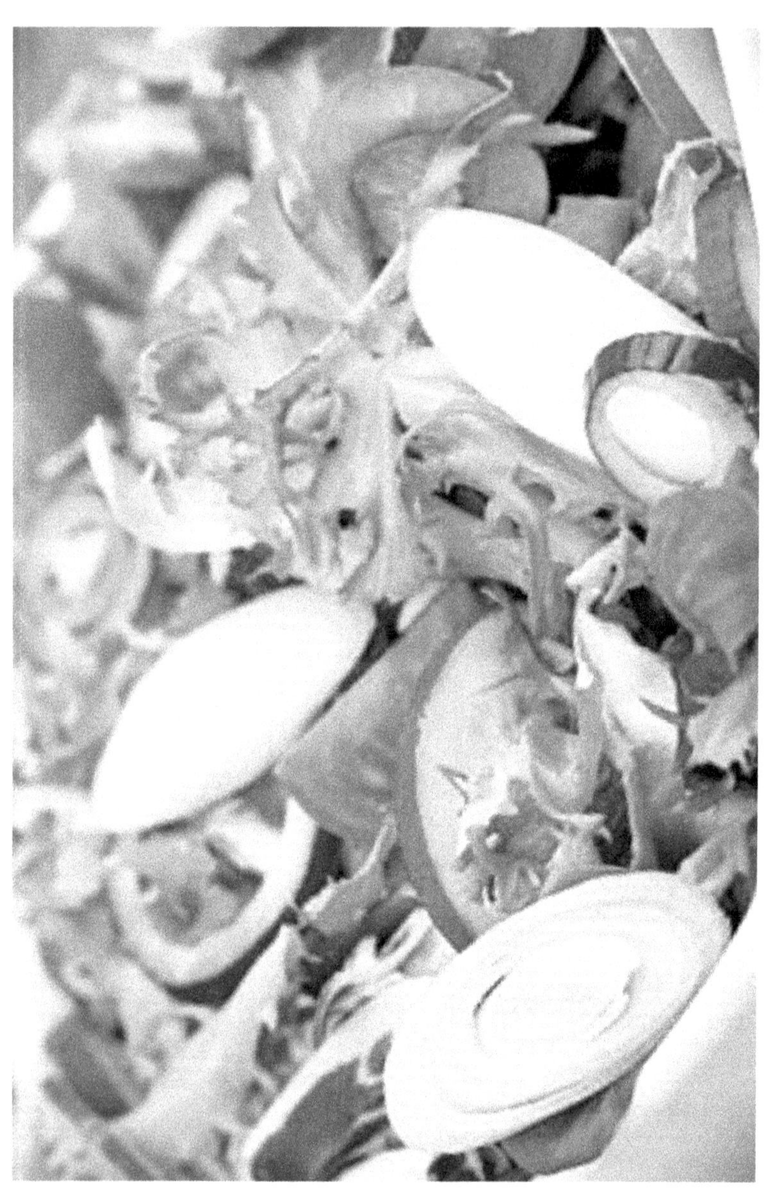

INTRODUCTION

The South Beach Diet Cookbook serves as a culinary companion to one of the most renowned and effective diet plans for achieving sustainable weight loss and promoting overall health. South Beach Diet revolutionized nutritional approaches by emphasizing the consumption of nutrient-dense, wholesome foods while steering clear of refined sugars and unhealthy fats. This cookbook is a treasure trove of flavorful recipes meticulously curated to align with the principles of the South Beach Diet. From delectable breakfast options to mouthwatering main courses and delightful desserts, this cookbook offers a diverse array of dishes that prioritize both taste and health. Whether you're a newcomer to the diet or a seasoned practitioner seeking culinary inspiration, the South Beach Diet Cookbook promises to transform your meals into delicious and nourishing creations, making healthy eating an enjoyable and satisfying journey.

South Beach Diet recipes offer a multitude of benefits that go beyond mere weight loss, promoting overall health and well-being through their unique approach to nutrition.

Weight Loss and Weight Management:

The recipes featured in the South Beach Diet Cookbook are designed to help individuals shed excess weight effectively and sustainably. By focusing on lean proteins, healthy fats, and low-glycemic carbohydrates, these recipes can aid in controlling hunger, reducing cravings, and facilitating healthy weight loss.

Balanced Nutrition:

The recipes emphasize the consumption of nutrient-dense foods, providing a balanced mix of macronutrients and essential vitamins and minerals. This balance supports overall health, boosts energy levels, and contributes to a sense of well-being.

Stable Blood Sugar Levels:

The South Beach Diet recipes utilize low-glycemic index (GI) foods that release glucose slowly into the bloodstream, helping to stabilize blood sugar levels. This approach can be particularly beneficial for individuals with diabetes or those seeking to manage blood sugar levels effectively.

Improved Heart Health:

With an emphasis on healthy fats, lean proteins, and whole grains, the South Beach Diet recipes align with heart-healthy eating patterns. By incorporating these recipes into your diet, you can potentially reduce the risk factors associated with heart disease, such as high cholesterol and high blood pressure.

Reduced Inflammation:

Many ingredients used in South Beach Diet recipes, such as leafy greens, fatty fish, nuts, and olive oil, possess anti-inflammatory properties. Consuming these foods can help combat inflammation in the body, potentially reducing the risk of chronic diseases linked to inflammation.

Enhanced Satiety and Energy:

The recipes prioritize fiber-rich foods, lean proteins, and healthy fats, which can contribute to increased feelings of fullness and sustained energy levels throughout the day. This can aid in controlling cravings and preventing overeating.

Versatility and Flavor:

Despite focusing on healthy and nutritious ingredients, the South Beach Diet recipes are far from bland. They offer a wide variety of flavorful options, showcasing the diversity and deliciousness of wholesome foods, making it easier to stick to a healthy eating plan.

CHAPTER ONE

21-Day South Beach Diet Meal Plan

DAYS	BREAKFAST	LUNCH	DINNER	SNACKS
1	Vegetable and feta cheese omelet.	Grilled chicken salad with mixed greens, tomatoes, and a vinaigrette dressing.	Baked salmon with roasted asparagus and quinoa.	Greek yogurt with berries, cucumber slices with hummus.
2	Spinach and tomato egg muffins.	Turkey and avocado lettuce wraps.	Zucchini noodles (zoodles) with lean ground turkey and marinara sauce.	Cottage cheese with sliced peaches, raw almonds.
3	Greek yogurt parfait with mixed fruits and nuts.	Tuna salad stuffed bell peppers.	Grilled shrimp with roasted Brussels sprouts and a side of brown rice.	Hard-boiled eggs, celery sticks with almond butter.
4	Veggie-packed omelet with mushrooms, bell peppers, and onions.	Grilled vegetable and chicken skewers.	Baked cod with steamed broccoli and a small portion of quinoa.	Almond butter with apple slices, cherry tomatoes with mozzarella cheese.
5	Greek yogurt with sliced almonds and a sprinkle of cinnamon.	Quinoa salad with black beans, corn, and grilled chicken.	Turkey meatballs in marinara sauce served with steamed	Carrot sticks with hummus, a small portion of mixed berries.

			cauliflower rice.	
6	Scrambled eggs with spinach and tomatoes.	Grilled salmon salad with mixed greens and a lemon vinaigrette.	Grilled chicken breast with roasted vegetables (bell peppers, zucchini, and onions).	Greek yogurt with a drizzle of honey, raw almonds.
7	Quinoa breakfast bowl with mixed fruits and nuts.	Turkey and vegetable stir-fry with a side of brown rice.	Baked turkey breast with green beans and a small sweet potato.	Cottage cheese with pineapple chunks, cucumber slices with tzatziki sauce.
8	Vegetable and cheese frittata.	Grilled chicken Caesar salad.	Baked salmon with steamed broccoli and a side of quinoa.	Greek yogurt with berries, carrot sticks with hummus.
9	Spinach and cheese scrambled eggs.	Turkey and avocado lettuce wraps.	Zucchini noodles with marinara sauce and lean ground turkey.	Cottage cheese with sliced peaches, raw almonds.
10	Greek yogurt parfait with mixed fruits and nuts.	Tuna salad stuffed bell peppers.	Grilled shrimp with roasted Brussels sprouts and a small portion of brown rice.	Hard-boiled eggs, celery sticks with almond butter.
11	Veggie and cheese omelet.	Grilled chicken salad with mixed greens and a	Baked salmon with roasted asparagus and a side of	Greek yogurt with berries, cucumber slices with hummus.

		vinaigrette dressing.	quinoa.
12	Spinach and tomato egg muffins.	Turkey and avocado lettuce wraps.	Zucchini noodles with lean ground turkey and marinara sauce.	Cottage cheese with sliced peaches, raw almonds.
13	Greek yogurt parfait with mixed fruits and nuts.	Tuna salad stuffed bell peppers.	Grilled shrimp with roasted Brussels sprouts and a small portion of brown rice.	Hard-boiled eggs, celery sticks with almond butter.
14	Vegetable and cheese frittata.	Grilled chicken Caesar salad.	Baked salmon with steamed broccoli and a side of quinoa.	Greek yogurt with berries, carrot sticks with hummus.
15	Spinach and cheese scrambled eggs.	Turkey and avocado lettuce wraps.	Zucchini noodles with marinara sauce and lean ground turkey.	Cottage cheese with sliced peaches, raw almonds.
16	Greek yogurt parfait with mixed fruits and nuts.	Tuna salad stuffed bell peppers.	Grilled shrimp with roasted Brussels sprouts and a small portion of brown rice.	Hard-boiled eggs, celery sticks with almond butter.
17	Veggie and cheese omelet.	Grilled chicken salad with mixed greens and a vinaigrette dressing.	Baked salmon with roasted asparagus and a side of quinoa.	Greek yogurt with berries, cucumber slices with hummus.
18	Spinach and	Turkey and	Zucchini	Cottage

	tomato egg muffins.	avocado lettuce wraps.	noodles with lean ground turkey and marinara sauce.	cheese with sliced peaches, raw almonds.
19	Vegetable and cheese frittata.	Grilled chicken Caesar salad.	Baked salmon with steamed broccoli and a side of quinoa.	Greek yogurt with berries, carrot sticks with hummus.
20	Spinach and cheese scrambled eggs.	Turkey and avocado lettuce wraps.	Zucchini noodles with marinara sauce and lean ground turkey.	Cottage cheese with sliced peaches, raw almonds.
21	Greek yogurt parfait with mixed fruits and nuts.	Tuna salad stuffed bell peppers.	Grilled shrimp with roasted Brussels sprouts and a small portion of brown rice.	Hard-boiled eggs, celery sticks with almond butter.

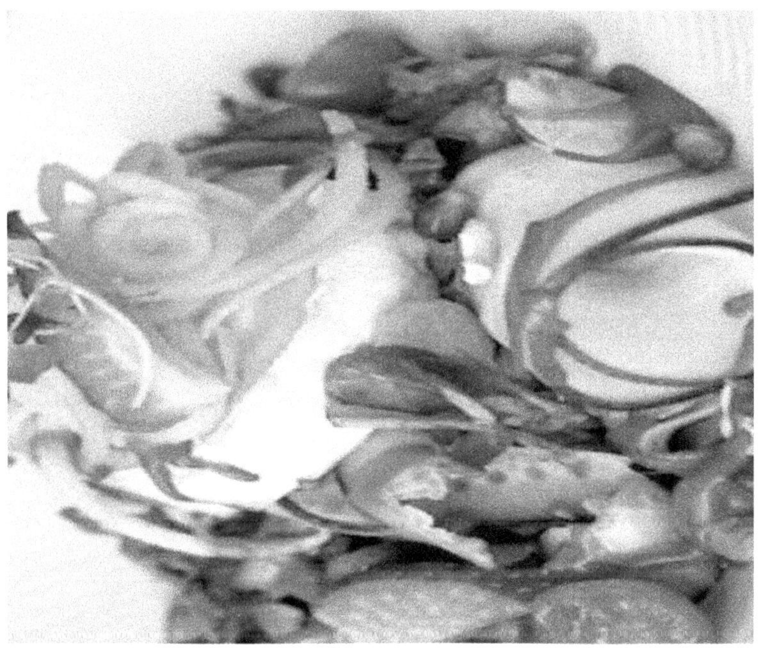

CHAPTER TWO

Grilled Lemon Herb Chicken

Ingredients:

- 4 boneless, skinless chicken breasts

- 2 tablespoons olive oil

- 2 cloves garlic, minced

- 2 tablespoons chopped fresh herbs (rosemary, thyme, or parsley)

- Zest and juice of 1 lemon

- Salt and pepper to taste

Preparation:

1. In a bowl, mix olive oil, garlic, herbs, lemon zest, lemon juice, salt, and pepper.

2. Marinate chicken breasts in the mixture for 30 minutes to 1 hour.

3. Preheat grill or stovetop grill pan over medium-high heat.

4. Grill chicken for 6-8 minutes per side or until fully cooked.

Baked Salmon with Dill Sauce

Ingredients:

- 4 salmon fillets

- 2 tablespoons olive oil

- Salt and pepper to taste

- 1/4 cup plain Greek yogurt

- 2 tablespoons chopped fresh dill

- 1 tablespoon lemon juice

- 1 teaspoon Dijon mustard

Preparation:

1. Preheat oven to 375°F (190°C).

2. Brush salmon fillets with olive oil and season with salt and pepper.

3. Place salmon on a baking sheet and bake for 12-15 minutes or until cooked through.

4. In a bowl, mix Greek yogurt, dill, lemon juice, and Dijon mustard for the sauce.

5. Serve baked salmon with the dill sauce on top.

Turkey and Vegetable Stir-Fry

Ingredients:

- 1 lb lean ground turkey

- 2 cups mixed vegetables (bell peppers, broccoli, carrots)

- 2 cloves garlic, minced

- 2 tablespoons low-sodium soy sauce

- 1 tablespoon olive oil

- Salt and pepper to taste

Preparation:

1. Heat olive oil in a large skillet over medium heat.

2. Add ground turkey and cook until browned.

3. Add minced garlic and mixed vegetables to the skillet, sauté for 5-7 minutes.

4. Stir in soy sauce, salt, and pepper, and cook for an additional 2-3 minutes.

Zucchini Noodles with Pesto Shrimp

Ingredients:

- 1 lb large shrimp, peeled and deveined

- 4 medium zucchinis, spiralized into noodles

- 1/4 cup basil pesto

- 2 tablespoons olive oil

- Salt and pepper to taste

- Grated Parmesan cheese (optional, for garnish)

Preparation:

1. In a bowl, toss shrimp with olive oil, salt, and pepper.

2. Heat a skillet over medium-high heat and cook shrimp for 2-3 minutes per side until pink and cooked through.

3. In the same skillet, add zucchini noodles and cook for 2-3 minutes until tender.

4. Toss zucchini noodles with pesto and top with cooked shrimp. Optionally, sprinkle with grated Parmesan cheese.

Baked Chicken with Tomato and Olive Relish
Ingredients:

- 4 boneless, skinless chicken breasts

- 1 cup cherry tomatoes, halved

- 1/4 cup Kalamata olives, chopped

- 2 tablespoons chopped fresh parsley

- 2 tablespoons olive oil

- 2 cloves garlic, minced

- Salt and pepper to taste

Preparation:

1. Preheat oven to 375°F (190°C).

2. Season chicken breasts with salt and pepper and place in a baking dish.

3. In a bowl, mix cherry tomatoes, olives, parsley, olive oil, minced garlic, salt, and pepper.

4. Spoon the tomato and olive mixture over the chicken breasts.

5. Bake for 20-25 minutes or until the chicken is fully cooked.

Cauliflower Fried Rice with Shrimp

Ingredients:

- 1 lb shrimp, peeled and deveined

- 4 cups cauliflower rice

- 1 cup mixed vegetables (peas, carrots, bell peppers)

- 2 cloves garlic, minced

- 2 tablespoons low-sodium soy sauce

- 1 tablespoon sesame oil

- 2 eggs, beaten

- Salt and pepper to taste

- Green onions (optional, for garnish)

Preparation:

1. Heat sesame oil in a large skillet or wok over medium-high heat.

2. Add shrimp and cook for 2-3 minutes until pink. Remove shrimp from the skillet.

3. In the same skillet, add garlic and mixed vegetables, sauté for 3-4 minutes.

4. Push vegetables to one side of the skillet and pour beaten eggs into the other side. Scramble the eggs until cooked.

5. Add cauliflower rice, cooked shrimp, and soy sauce to the skillet. Stir-fry for 5-6 minutes until heated through.

6. Season with salt and pepper, garnish with chopped green onions if desired.

Baked Cod with Herbed Tomato Salsa

Ingredients:

- 4 cod fillets

- 2 cups cherry tomatoes, halved

- 2 tablespoons chopped fresh basil

- 2 tablespoons chopped fresh parsley

- 2 tablespoons olive oil

- 2 cloves garlic, minced

- Salt and pepper to taste

- Lemon wedges (for serving)

Preparation:

1. Preheat oven to 375°F (190°C).

2. Place cod fillets in a baking dish and season with salt and pepper.

3. In a bowl, mix cherry tomatoes, basil, parsley, olive oil, minced garlic, salt, and pepper.

4. Spoon the tomato mixture over the cod fillets.

5. Bake for 15-20 minutes or until the cod is flaky and cooked through.

6. Serve with lemon wedges.

Turkey and Black Bean Chili

Ingredients:

- 1 lb ground turkey

- 1 can (15 oz) black beans, drained and rinsed

- 1 can (14 oz) diced tomatoes

- 1 onion, diced

- 2 cloves garlic, minced

- 1 tablespoon chili powder

- 1 teaspoon ground cumin

- 1 teaspoon paprika

- Salt and pepper to taste

- Chopped cilantro (optional, for garnish)

Preparation:

1. In a large pot or Dutch oven, cook ground turkey over medium heat until browned.

2. Add diced onion and minced garlic, cook for 2-3 minutes.

3. Stir in chili powder, cumin, paprika, salt, and pepper.

4. Add diced tomatoes and black beans to the pot. Bring to a simmer and let it cook for 15-20 minutes.

5. Serve the turkey and black bean chili hot, garnished with chopped cilantro if desired.

Eggplant and Turkey Lasagna

Ingredients:

- 1 large eggplant, sliced lengthwise

- 1 lb ground turkey

- 2 cups marinara sauce (look for low-sugar or homemade)

- 1 cup part-skim ricotta cheese

- 1 cup shredded mozzarella cheese

- 1/4 cup grated Parmesan cheese

- 1 teaspoon Italian seasoning

- Salt and pepper to taste

- Fresh basil leaves (for garnish)

Preparation:

1. Preheat oven to 375°F (190°C).

2. Lightly salt eggplant slices and let them sit for
   15 minutes. Pat dry with paper towels.

3. In a skillet, cook ground turkey until browned.
   Add marinara sauce and Italian seasoning,
   simmer for 5-7 minutes.

4. In a separate bowl, mix ricotta cheese, half of
   the mozzarella cheese, and grated Parmesan
   cheese.

5. In a baking dish, layer marinara sauce with
   turkey, eggplant slices, and cheese mixture.
   Repeat the layers.

6. Top with the remaining mozzarella cheese.

7. Cover with foil and bake for 25 minutes.
   Uncover and bake for an additional 10 minutes
   until the cheese is golden and bubbly.

8. Garnish with fresh basil leaves before serving.

Grilled Vegetable and Chicken Skewers
Ingredients:

- 1 lb boneless, skinless chicken breasts, cut into
  cubes

- 2 bell peppers (red, yellow, or green), cut into
  chunks

- 1 zucchini, sliced

- 1 red onion, cut into chunks

- 2 tablespoons olive oil

- 2 cloves garlic, minced

- 1 teaspoon dried oregano

- Salt and pepper to taste

- Wooden skewers, soaked in water for 30 minutes

Preparation:

1. Preheat grill or grill pan over medium-high heat.

2. In a bowl, mix olive oil, minced garlic, dried oregano, salt, and pepper.

3. Thread chicken cubes, bell peppers, zucchini slices, and onion chunks onto the soaked skewers.

4. Brush the skewers with the olive oil mixture.

5. Grill skewers for 8-10 minutes, turning occasionally, until chicken is cooked through and vegetables are charred and tender.

CHAPTER THREE

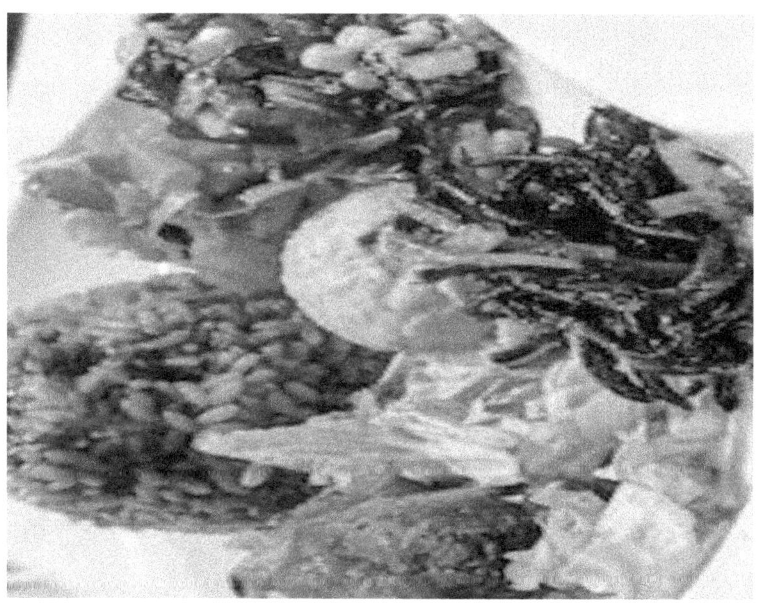

Cucumber Avocado Salsa

Ingredients:

- 1 ripe avocado, diced

- 1 cucumber, diced

- 1 tomato, diced

- 1/4 red onion, finely chopped

- 2 tablespoons chopped cilantro

- Juice of 1 lime

- Salt and pepper to taste

Preparation:

1. In a bowl, combine diced avocado, cucumber, tomato, red onion, and cilantro.

2. Squeeze lime juice over the mixture and gently toss to combine.

3. Season with salt and pepper. Serve with whole grain tortilla chips or cucumber slices.

Greek Yogurt Veggie Dip
Ingredients:

- 1 cup plain Greek yogurt

- 1 teaspoon dried dill

- 1/2 teaspoon garlic powder

- 1/2 teaspoon onion powder

- Salt and pepper to taste

- Assorted vegetable sticks (carrots, celery, bell peppers) for dipping

Preparation:

1. In a bowl, mix Greek yogurt, dried dill, garlic powder, onion powder, salt, and pepper until well combined.

2. Chill in the refrigerator for at least 30 minutes before serving with vegetable sticks.

Spicy Roasted Chickpeas

Ingredients:

- 1 can (15 oz) chickpeas, drained and rinsed

- 1 tablespoon olive oil

- 1 teaspoon paprika

- 1/2 teaspoon cayenne pepper

- 1/2 teaspoon garlic powder

- Salt to taste

Preparation:

1. Preheat oven to 400°F (200°C).

2. Pat dry the chickpeas with a paper towel to remove excess moisture.

3. In a bowl, toss chickpeas with olive oil, paprika, cayenne pepper, garlic powder, and salt.

4. Spread chickpeas on a baking sheet and bake for 25-30 minutes until crispy.

5. Let them cool before serving as a crunchy snack.

Caprese Salad Skewers

Ingredients:

- Cherry tomatoes

- Fresh mozzarella cheese, cut into cubes

- Fresh basil leaves

- Balsamic glaze (optional)

- Toothpicks or small skewers

Preparation:

1. Thread a cherry tomato, a cube of mozzarella, and a basil leaf onto each toothpick or skewer.

2. Arrange the skewers on a serving platter.

3. Drizzle with balsamic glaze if desired before serving.

Egg Salad Cucumber Bites

Ingredients:

- 3 hard-boiled eggs, peeled and chopped

- 2 tablespoons plain Greek yogurt

- 1 tablespoon Dijon mustard

- 1 tablespoon finely chopped chives or green onions

- Salt and pepper to taste

- English cucumber, sliced into rounds

Preparation:

1. In a bowl, mix chopped hard-boiled eggs, Greek yogurt, Dijon mustard, chopped chives, salt, and pepper until well combined.

2. Place a spoonful of egg salad on each cucumber round. Serve chilled.

Smoked Salmon Roll-Ups

Ingredients:

- Smoked salmon slices

- Cream cheese or Greek yogurt cream cheese

- Cucumber strips

- Fresh dill (optional)

Preparation:

1. Spread a thin layer of cream cheese on each smoked salmon slice.

2. Place a cucumber strip at one end and roll up the salmon slice.

3. Secure with a toothpick and garnish with fresh dill if desired. Serve chilled.

Stuffed Bell Pepper Poppers

Ingredients:

- Mini bell peppers, halved and seeded

- 1/2 cup low-fat cream cheese

- 1/4 cup chopped fresh parsley

- 1/4 cup chopped sun-dried tomatoes (packed in olive oil)

- Salt and pepper to taste

Preparation:

1. In a bowl, mix cream cheese, chopped parsley, sun-dried tomatoes, salt, and pepper.

2. Spoon the cream cheese mixture into each halved bell pepper.

3. Serve as is or bake at 375°F (190°C) for 10-12 minutes until peppers are tender and cheese is slightly melted.

Zucchini Hummus

Ingredients:

- 2 medium zucchinis, chopped

- 2 cloves garlic, minced

- 2 tablespoons tahini

- 2 tablespoons olive oil

- Juice of 1 lemon

- Salt and pepper to taste

- Pinch of cumin (optional)

- Vegetable sticks or whole grain crackers for dipping

Preparation:

1. Steam or boil chopped zucchinis until tender. Drain and let cool.

2. In a food processor, blend cooked zucchinis, minced garlic, tahini, olive oil, lemon juice, salt, pepper, and cumin until smooth.

3. Adjust seasoning if needed. Serve with vegetable sticks or crackers.

Turkey Lettuce Wraps
Ingredients:

- Romaine lettuce leaves

- 1 lb ground turkey

- 2 cloves garlic, minced

- 1 tablespoon low-sodium soy sauce

- 1 teaspoon sesame oil

- 1/2 cup shredded carrots

- 1/2 cup chopped water chestnuts (canned, drained)

- Green onions, chopped (for garnish)

Preparation:

1. Heat sesame oil in a skillet over medium heat. Add minced garlic and ground turkey, cook until browned.

2. Stir in soy sauce, shredded carrots, and chopped water chestnuts. Cook for another 3-4 minutes.

3. Spoon the turkey mixture onto romaine lettuce leaves, garnish with chopped green onions, and serve.

Baked Parmesan Zucchini Chips

Ingredients:

- 2 medium zucchinis, thinly sliced

- 1/2 cup grated Parmesan cheese

- 1 teaspoon garlic powder

- 1 teaspoon paprika

- Salt and pepper to taste

- Cooking spray

Preparation:

1. Preheat oven to 425°F (220°C). Line a baking sheet with parchment paper and coat it with cooking spray.

2. In a bowl, combine grated Parmesan cheese, garlic powder, paprika, salt, and pepper.

3. Coat each zucchini slice with the Parmesan mixture and place them on the prepared baking sheet.

4. Bake for 15-20 minutes until the zucchini chips are golden and crispy.

CHAPTER FOUR

Whole Grain Recipes For South Beach Diet

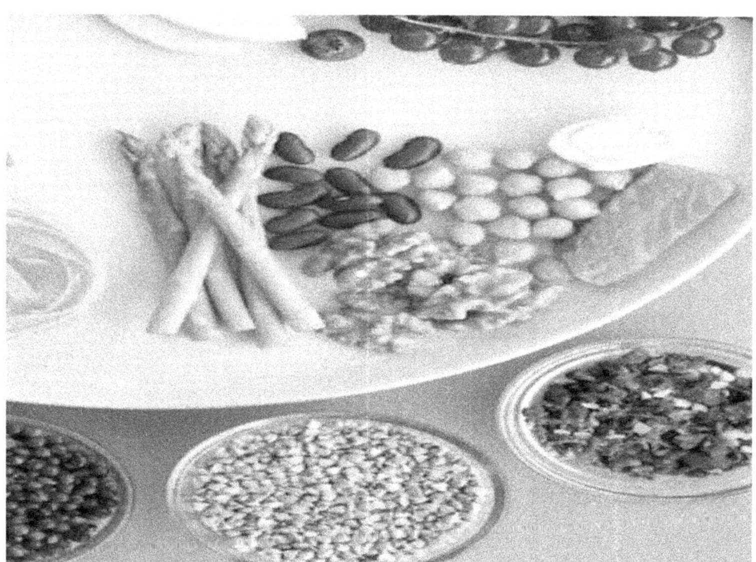

Quinoa Salad

Ingredients:

- 1 cup quinoa, rinsed

- 2 cups water or low-sodium vegetable broth

- 1 cucumber, diced

- 1 bell pepper (any color), diced

- 1/4 red onion, finely chopped

- 1/4 cup chopped fresh parsley

- Juice of 1 lemon

- 2 tablespoons olive oil

- Salt and pepper to taste

Preparation:

1. In a saucepan, combine quinoa and water or vegetable broth. Bring to a boil, then reduce heat and simmer covered for 15-20 minutes until quinoa is cooked and liquid is absorbed. Let it cool.

2. In a large bowl, combine cooked quinoa, diced cucumber, bell pepper, red onion, and chopped parsley.

3. In a small bowl, whisk together lemon juice, olive oil, salt, and pepper. Pour over the quinoa mixture and toss to combine. Serve chilled.

Whole Grain Veggie Wrap
Ingredients:

- Whole grain wraps or tortillas

- Hummus (store-bought or homemade)

- Sliced avocado

- Shredded carrots

- Sliced cucumbers

- Mixed salad greens

- Sprouts (optional)

- Sliced bell peppers

Preparation:

1. Spread a layer of hummus onto the whole grain wrap.

2. Layer sliced avocado, shredded carrots, cucumbers, salad greens, sprouts (if using), and bell peppers on top of the hummus.

3. Roll up the wrap tightly and cut in half. Serve as a nutritious and filling lunch or snack.

Brown Rice Stuffed Bell Peppers
Ingredients:

- 4 bell peppers (any color), tops removed and seeds removed

- 1 cup cooked brown rice

- 1 can (15 oz) black beans, drained and rinsed

- 1 cup corn kernels (fresh, canned, or frozen)

- 1 cup diced tomatoes

- 1/2 cup diced onion

- 1 teaspoon chili powder

- 1/2 teaspoon cumin

- Salt and pepper to taste

- Shredded cheese (optional, for topping)

Preparation:

1. Preheat oven to 375°F (190°C).

2. In a bowl, mix cooked brown rice, black beans, corn kernels, diced tomatoes, diced onion, chili powder, cumin, salt, and pepper.

3. Spoon the rice mixture into each bell pepper.

4. Place stuffed peppers in a baking dish and cover with foil. Bake for 25-30 minutes or until peppers are tender.

5. Optionally, sprinkle shredded cheese on top and bake for an additional 5 minutes until cheese is melted.

Whole Wheat Pasta Primavera

Ingredients:

- 8 oz whole wheat pasta (penne or spaghetti)

- 2 tablespoons olive oil

- 2 cloves garlic, minced

- 1 cup broccoli florets

- 1 cup sliced bell peppers

- 1 cup sliced zucchini

- 1 cup cherry tomatoes, halved

- 1/4 cup chopped fresh basil

- Salt and pepper to taste

- Grated Parmesan cheese (optional, for garnish)

Preparation:

1. Cook whole wheat pasta according to package instructions. Drain and set aside.

2. Heat olive oil in a large skillet over medium heat. Add minced garlic and sauté for 1 minute.

3. Add broccoli florets, sliced bell peppers, and sliced zucchini to the skillet. Cook for 5-7 minutes until vegetables are tender.

4. Stir in cherry tomatoes, cooked pasta, chopped basil, salt, and pepper. Toss everything together until heated through.

5. Serve the pasta primavera with optional grated Parmesan cheese on top.

Farro Salad with Roasted Vegetables

Ingredients:

- 1 cup farro, rinsed

- 3 cups water or vegetable broth

- 1 red bell pepper, sliced

- 1 yellow bell pepper, sliced

- 1 zucchini, sliced

- 1 yellow squash, sliced

- 1 red onion, sliced

- 2 tablespoons olive oil

- 2 tablespoons balsamic vinegar

- 2 cloves garlic, minced

- Salt and pepper to taste

- Chopped fresh herbs (such as parsley or basil) for garnish

Preparation:

1. Preheat oven to 400°F (200°C).

2. In a saucepan, combine farro and water or vegetable broth. Bring to a boil, then reduce heat and simmer covered for 25-30 minutes until farro is tender. Drain any excess liquid and let it cool.

3. On a baking sheet, spread out sliced bell peppers, zucchini, yellow squash, and red onion. Drizzle with olive oil and balsamic vinegar, sprinkle minced garlic, salt, and pepper. Toss to coat.

4. Roast vegetables in the preheated oven for 20-25 minutes until tender and slightly caramelized.

5. In a large bowl, mix cooked farro and roasted vegetables. Garnish with chopped fresh herbs before serving.

Barley and Vegetable Soup

Ingredients:

- 1 cup pearl barley

- 6 cups low-sodium vegetable broth

- 2 tablespoons olive oil

- 1 onion, diced

- 2 carrots, diced

- 2 celery stalks, diced

- 2 cloves garlic, minced

- 1 can (14 oz) diced tomatoes

- 1 teaspoon dried thyme

- Salt and pepper to taste

- Chopped fresh parsley (optional, for garnish)

Preparation:

1. Rinse pearl barley under cold water.

2. In a large pot, heat olive oil over medium heat. Add diced onion, carrots, celery, and minced garlic. Sauté for 5-7 minutes until vegetables are tender.

3. Add rinsed barley, vegetable broth, diced tomatoes (with juices), dried thyme, salt, and pepper to the pot. Bring to a boil, then reduce heat and simmer covered for 40-45 minutes until barley is cooked through.

4. Adjust seasoning if needed. Serve the barley and vegetable soup hot, garnished with chopped fresh parsley if desired.

Whole Grain Pita Bread Pizza

Ingredients:

- Whole grain pita bread rounds

- Tomato sauce or marinara sauce (low-sugar)

- Shredded part-skim mozzarella cheese

- Assorted toppings (sliced tomatoes, bell peppers, mushrooms, spinach, etc.)

- Dried oregano or Italian seasoning

Preparation:

1. Preheat oven to 375°F (190°C).

2. Place whole grain pita bread rounds on a baking sheet.

3. Spread a thin layer of tomato or marinara sauce on each pita round.

4. Sprinkle shredded mozzarella cheese and add your choice of toppings.

5. Sprinkle dried oregano or Italian seasoning on top.

6. Bake in the preheated oven for 10-12 minutes until cheese is melted and bubbly.

Bulgur Salad with Chickpeas and Herbs
Ingredients:

- 1 cup bulgur wheat

- 2 cups water or vegetable broth

- 1 can (15 oz) chickpeas, drained and rinsed

- 1 cucumber, diced

- 1 red bell pepper, diced

- 1/4 cup chopped fresh parsley

- 1/4 cup chopped fresh mint

- Juice of 1 lemon

- 2 tablespoons olive oil

- Salt and pepper to taste

Preparation:

1. In a saucepan, combine bulgur wheat and water or vegetable broth. Bring to a boil, then reduce heat and simmer covered for 10-12 minutes until bulgur is cooked. Let it cool.

2. In a large bowl, mix cooked bulgur wheat, chickpeas, diced cucumber, diced bell pepper, chopped parsley, chopped mint, lemon juice, olive oil, salt, and pepper.

3. Toss everything together until well combined. Serve the bulgur salad chilled.

Whole Grain Breakfast Burrito

Ingredients:

- Whole grain tortillas or wraps

- 4 eggs, beaten

- 1/2 cup black beans, drained and rinsed

- 1/4 cup diced bell peppers

- 1/4 cup diced tomatoes

- 2 tablespoons chopped cilantro

- 1/2 cup shredded part-skim mozzarella cheese

- Salt and pepper to taste

- Salsa (optional, for serving)

Preparation:

1. In a skillet over medium heat, scramble beaten eggs until cooked through.

2. Add black beans, diced bell peppers, diced tomatoes, chopped cilantro, shredded mozzarella cheese, salt, and pepper to the skillet. Cook for an additional 2-3 minutes until heated through.

3. Warm whole grain tortillas or wraps. Spoon the egg and vegetable mixture onto each tortilla and roll it up.

4. Serve breakfast burritos with salsa if desired.

Whole Wheat Couscous with Roasted Vegetables
Ingredients:

- 1 cup whole wheat couscous

- 1 1/4 cups low-sodium vegetable broth

- 1 zucchini, diced

- 1 yellow squash, diced

- 1 red onion, diced

- 1 red bell pepper, diced

- 2 tablespoons olive oil

- 1 teaspoon dried oregano

- 1 teaspoon paprika

- Salt and pepper to taste

Preparation:

1. Preheat oven to 400°F (200°C).

2. In a baking dish, toss diced zucchini, yellow squash, red onion, and red bell pepper with olive oil, dried oregano, paprika, salt, and pepper.

3. Roast vegetables in the preheated oven for 20-
    25 minutes until tender and slightly golden.

4. In a saucepan, bring vegetable broth to a boil.
    Remove from heat and stir in whole wheat
    couscous. Cover and let it sit for 5 minutes until
    couscous absorbs the liquid.

5. Fluff the couscous with a fork and serve with
    roasted vegetables on top.

CHAPTER FIVE

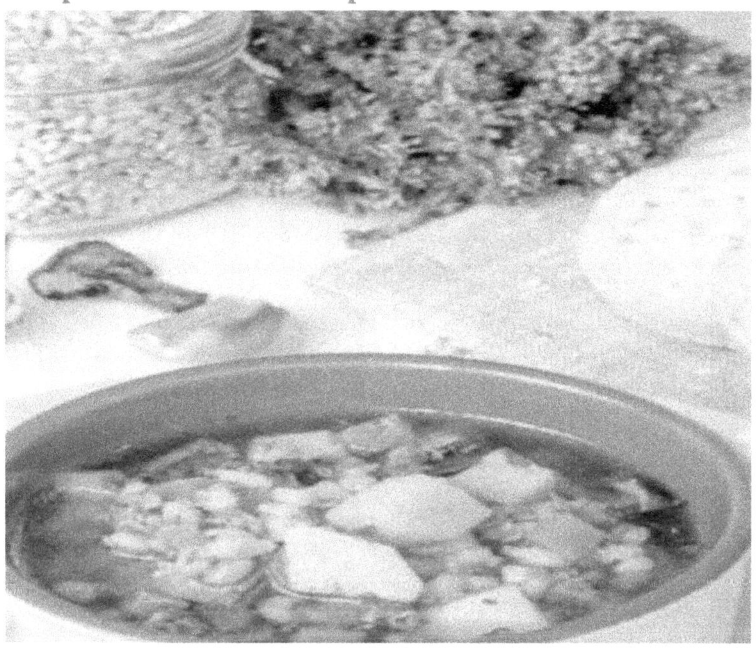

Tomato Basil Soup

Ingredients:

- 6 tomatoes, chopped

- 1 onion, chopped

- 3 cloves garlic, minced

- 2 cups low-sodium vegetable broth

- 1/4 cup chopped fresh basil

- 2 tablespoons olive oil

- Salt and pepper to taste

Preparation:

1. Heat olive oil in a pot over medium heat. Add chopped onion and garlic, sauté for 2-3 minutes until fragrant.

2. Add chopped tomatoes and cook for another 5 minutes until tomatoes soften.

3. Pour in vegetable broth, bring to a boil, then reduce heat and simmer for 15-20 minutes.

4. Blend the soup using an immersion blender or transfer to a blender to puree until smooth.

5. Stir in chopped basil, salt, and pepper. Serve hot.

Lentil Vegetable Soup

Ingredients:

- 1 cup dried green or brown lentils, rinsed

- 6 cups low-sodium vegetable broth

- 1 onion, chopped

- 2 carrots, diced

- 2 celery stalks, diced

- 1 can (14 oz) diced tomatoes

- 2 cloves garlic, minced

- 1 teaspoon ground cumin

- 1 teaspoon paprika

- Salt and pepper to taste

- Chopped fresh parsley (optional, for garnish)

Preparation:

1. In a large pot, combine lentils, vegetable broth, chopped onion, diced carrots, diced celery, diced tomatoes (with juices), minced garlic, ground cumin, paprika, salt, and pepper.

2. Bring to a boil, then reduce heat and simmer covered for 25-30 minutes until lentils and vegetables are tender.

3. Adjust seasoning if needed. Garnish with chopped fresh parsley before serving.

Spinach and White Bean Soup

Ingredients:

- 1 tablespoon olive oil

- 1 onion, chopped

- 2 cloves garlic, minced

- 4 cups low-sodium vegetable broth

- 2 cans (15 oz each) cannellini beans, drained and rinsed

- 4 cups fresh spinach leaves

- 1 teaspoon dried thyme

- Salt and pepper to taste

- Grated Parmesan cheese (optional, for garnish)

Preparation:

1. Heat olive oil in a pot over medium heat. Add chopped onion and minced garlic, sauté for 2-3 minutes until softened.

2. Pour in vegetable broth and bring to a simmer.

3. Add cannellini beans, fresh spinach leaves, dried thyme, salt, and pepper. Cook for 5-7 minutes until spinach wilts.

4. Use an immersion blender to partially blend the soup for a thicker consistency (optional).

5. Serve the soup hot, garnished with grated Parmesan cheese if desired.

Butternut Squash Soup

Ingredients:

- 1 medium butternut squash, peeled, seeded, and cubed

- 1 onion, chopped

- 2 cloves garlic, minced

- 4 cups low-sodium vegetable broth

- 1 teaspoon ground cumin

- 1/2 teaspoon ground cinnamon

- 2 tablespoons olive oil

- Salt and pepper to taste

- Pumpkin seeds (optional, for garnish)

Preparation:

1. Preheat oven to 400°F (200°C). Place butternut squash cubes on a baking sheet, drizzle with olive oil, and season with salt and pepper. Roast for 25-30 minutes until tender.

2. In a pot, heat olive oil over medium heat. Add chopped onion and minced garlic, sauté for 2-3 minutes until softened.

3. Add roasted butternut squash, vegetable broth, ground cumin, ground cinnamon, salt, and pepper. Bring to a boil, then reduce heat and simmer for 15-20 minutes.

4. Use an immersion blender or transfer to a blender to puree until smooth.

5. Serve the butternut squash soup hot, garnished with pumpkin seeds if desired.

Chicken and Vegetable Soup

Ingredients:

- 1 lb boneless, skinless chicken breasts

- 6 cups low-sodium chicken broth

- 1 onion, chopped

- 2 carrots, sliced

- 2 celery stalks, sliced

- 1 cup green beans, trimmed and chopped

- 1 can (14 oz) diced tomatoes

- 2 cloves garlic, minced

- 1 teaspoon dried thyme

- Salt and pepper to taste

- Chopped fresh parsley (optional, for garnish)

Preparation:

1. In a large pot, bring chicken broth to a boil. Add boneless, skinless chicken breasts and cook for 15-20 minutes until chicken is cooked through. Remove chicken from the pot and shred using forks.

2. To the same pot with broth, add chopped onion, sliced carrots, sliced celery, chopped green beans, diced tomatoes (with juices), minced garlic, dried thyme, salt, and pepper.

3. Simmer for 15-20 minutes until vegetables are tender.

4. Return shredded chicken to the pot and cook for an additional 5 minutes.

5. Garnish the chicken and vegetable soup with chopped fresh parsley before serving.

Mediterranean Quinoa Salad

Ingredients:

- 1 cup quinoa, cooked and cooled

- 1 cucumber, diced

- 1 cup cherry tomatoes, halved

- 1/4 cup chopped red onion

- 1/4 cup chopped fresh parsley

- 1/4 cup chopped fresh mint

- Juice of 1 lemon

- 2 tablespoons olive oil

- Salt and pepper to taste

- Feta cheese crumbles (optional, for garnish)

Preparation:

1. In a large bowl, combine cooked quinoa, diced cucumber, halved cherry tomatoes, chopped red onion, chopped parsley, and chopped mint.

2. In a small bowl, whisk together lemon juice, olive oil, salt, and pepper. Pour over the salad and toss to combine.

3. Top with feta cheese crumbles if desired before serving.

Kale and Chickpea Salad

Ingredients:

- 4 cups chopped kale leaves (ribs removed)

- 1 can (15 oz) chickpeas, drained and rinsed

- 1/4 cup grated Parmesan cheese

- 1/4 cup sliced almonds

- 2 tablespoons lemon juice

- 2 tablespoons olive oil

- 1 clove garlic, minced

- Salt and pepper to taste

Preparation:

1. In a large bowl, massage chopped kale leaves with lemon juice and olive oil for a few minutes to soften.

2. Add drained and rinsed chickpeas, grated Parmesan cheese, sliced almonds, minced garlic, salt, and pepper. Toss everything together until well combined.

3. Serve the kale and chickpea salad immediately or let it sit for 10-15 minutes for flavors to meld.

Greek Salad

Ingredients:

- 2 cups chopped romaine lettuce

- 1 cucumber, diced

- 1 cup cherry tomatoes, halved

- 1/4 cup sliced red onion

- 1/4 cup sliced Kalamata olives

- 1/2 cup crumbled feta cheese

- 2 tablespoons olive oil

- 2 tablespoons red wine vinegar

- 1 teaspoon dried oregano

- Salt and pepper to taste

Preparation:

1. In a large bowl, combine chopped romaine lettuce, diced cucumber, halved cherry tomatoes, sliced red onion, sliced Kalamata olives, and crumbled feta cheese.

2. In a small bowl, whisk together olive oil, red wine vinegar, dried oregano, salt, and pepper. Drizzle over the salad and toss to coat.

3. Serve the Greek salad immediately as a refreshing side dish.

Grilled Chicken Caesar Salad

Ingredients:

- 2 boneless, skinless chicken breasts

- 4 cups chopped Romaine lettuce

- 1/4 cup grated Parmesan cheese

- Whole grain croutons

- Caesar dressing (store-bought or homemade)

- Olive oil

- Salt and pepper to taste

Preparation:

1. Preheat grill or grill pan over medium-high heat. Brush chicken breasts with olive oil, season with salt, and pepper. Grill for 6-8 minutes per side until fully cooked. Let it rest for a few minutes before slicing.

2. In a large bowl, toss chopped Romaine lettuce with Caesar dressing until well coated.

3. Divide dressed lettuce among plates. Top with grilled chicken slices, grated Parmesan cheese, and whole grain croutons.

Tuna and White Bean Salad

Ingredients:

- 2 cans (5 oz each) tuna in water, drained

- 1 can (15 oz) cannellini beans, drained and rinsed

- 1/2 red onion, finely chopped

- 1 celery stalk, finely chopped

- 1/4 cup chopped fresh parsley

- Juice of 1 lemon

- 2 tablespoons olive oil

- Salt and pepper to taste

Preparation:

1. In a large bowl, mix drained tuna, cannellini beans, finely chopped red onion, finely chopped celery, and chopped fresh parsley.

2. In a small bowl, whisk together lemon juice, olive oil, salt, and pepper. Pour over the salad and toss to combine.

3. Serve the tuna and white bean salad chilled.

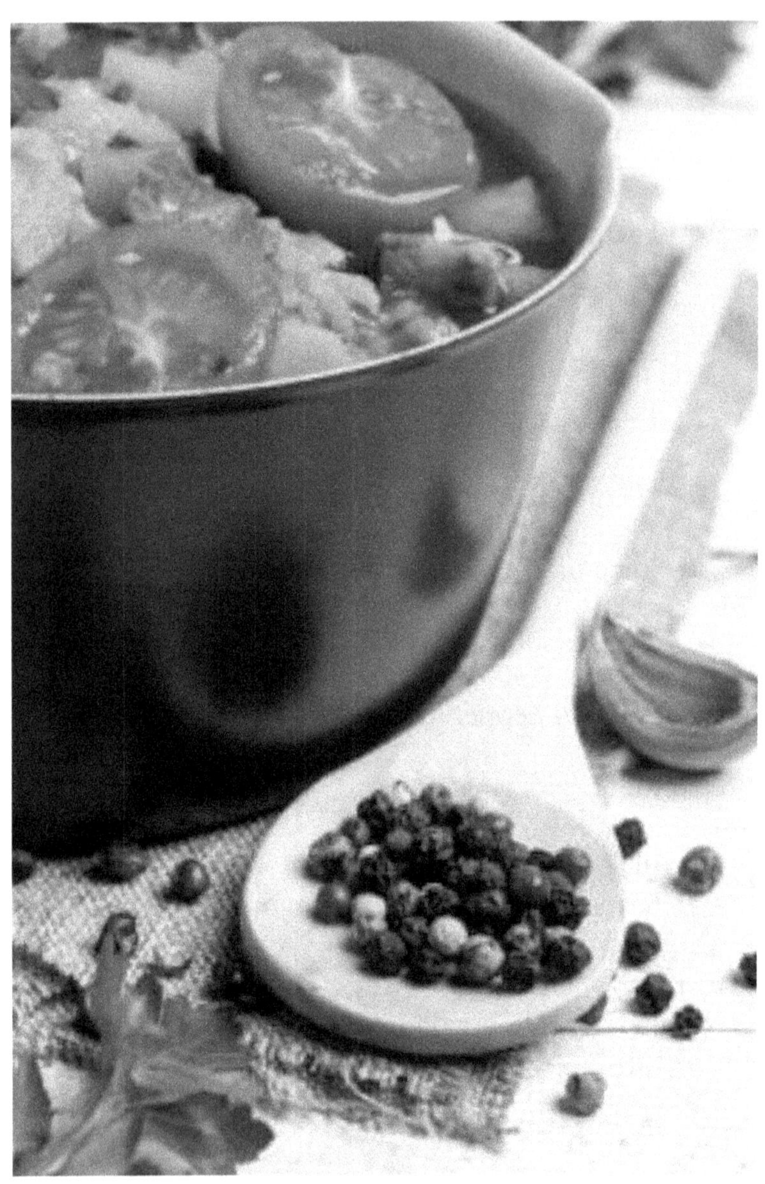

CHAPTER SIX

Sides And Desserts Recipes For South Beach Diet

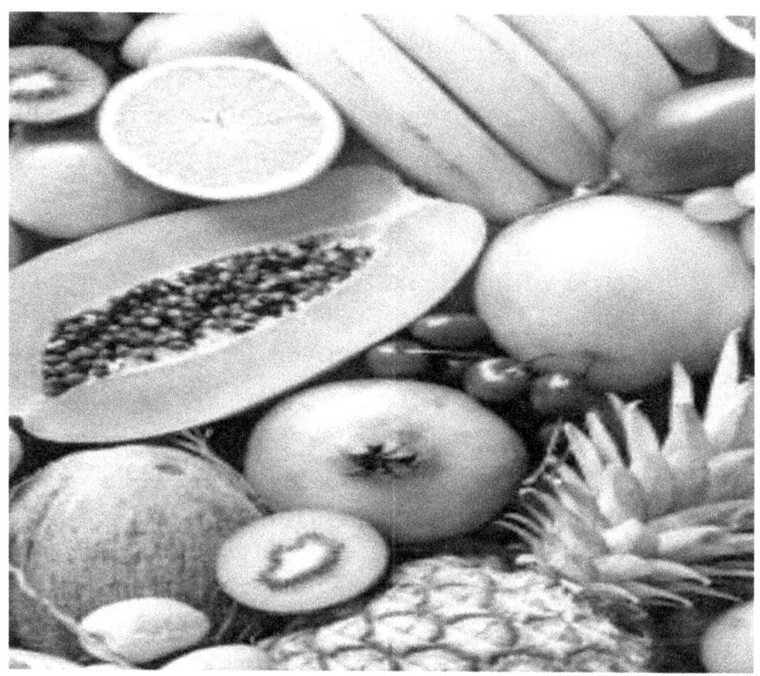

Garlic Roasted Asparagus

Ingredients:

- 1 bunch asparagus, tough ends trimmed

- 2 tablespoons olive oil

- 3 cloves garlic, minced

- Salt and pepper to taste

- Lemon wedges (optional, for serving)

Preparation:

1. Preheat oven to 400°F (200°C).

2. Place trimmed asparagus on a baking sheet. Drizzle with olive oil and minced garlic. Toss to coat evenly.

3. Season with salt and pepper.

4. Roast in the preheated oven for 12-15 minutes until asparagus is tender-crisp.

5. Squeeze fresh lemon juice over the roasted asparagus before serving (if desired).

Cauliflower "Rice" Stir-Fry

Ingredients:

- 1 head cauliflower, grated or processed into rice-like texture

- 1 tablespoon olive oil

- 2 cloves garlic, minced

- 1 cup mixed vegetables (bell peppers, broccoli, carrots, etc.), chopped

- 2 tablespoons low-sodium soy sauce or tamari

- 1 tablespoon sesame oil (optional)

- Salt and pepper to taste

- Chopped green onions (optional, for garnish)

Preparation:

1. In a large skillet or wok, heat olive oil over medium-high heat.

2. Add minced garlic and grated cauliflower "rice." Stir-fry for 3-4 minutes until cauliflower is slightly tender.

3. Add chopped mixed vegetables and continue stir-frying for another 3-4 minutes until vegetables are cooked but still crisp.

4. Pour in low-sodium soy sauce or tamari, and sesame oil (if using). Season with salt and pepper. Stir-fry for an additional minute.

5. Garnish with chopped green onions before serving.

Grilled Lemon Herb Zucchini

Ingredients:

- 2-3 medium zucchinis, sliced lengthwise into planks

- 2 tablespoons olive oil

- Juice of 1 lemon

- 2 cloves garlic, minced

- 1 tablespoon chopped fresh herbs (such as basil, parsley, or thyme)

- Salt and pepper to taste

Preparation:

1. Preheat grill or grill pan over medium-high heat.

2. In a bowl, whisk together olive oil, lemon juice, minced garlic, chopped fresh herbs, salt, and pepper.

3. Brush both sides of zucchini planks with the prepared mixture.

4. Grill zucchini planks for 3-4 minutes per side until grill marks appear and zucchini is tender.

5. Serve the grilled lemon herb zucchini hot as a flavorful side dish.

Spicy Roasted Brussels Sprouts

Ingredients:

- 1 lb Brussels sprouts, trimmed and halved

- 2 tablespoons olive oil

- 2 teaspoons paprika

- 1/2 teaspoon cayenne pepper (adjust to taste)

- Salt and pepper to taste

- Lemon wedges (optional, for serving)

Preparation:

1. Preheat oven to 400°F (200°C).

2. Toss trimmed and halved Brussels sprouts with olive oil, paprika, cayenne pepper, salt, and pepper in a mixing bowl.

3. Spread Brussels sprouts on a baking sheet in a single layer.

4. Roast in the preheated oven for 20-25 minutes until Brussels sprouts are crispy and browned.

5. Serve with optional lemon wedges for added zest if desired.

Baked Parmesan Zucchini Fries

Ingredients:

- 2 medium zucchinis, cut into sticks

- 1/2 cup grated Parmesan cheese

- 1/4 cup almond flour or whole wheat breadcrumbs

- 1 teaspoon garlic powder

- 1 teaspoon paprika

- Salt and pepper to taste

- Cooking spray

Preparation:

1. Preheat oven to 425°F (220°C). Line a baking sheet with parchment paper and coat it with cooking spray.

2. In a shallow bowl, combine grated Parmesan cheese, almond flour or breadcrumbs, garlic powder, paprika, salt, and pepper.

3. Dip zucchini sticks into the Parmesan mixture, pressing gently to coat.

4. Place coated zucchini sticks on the prepared baking sheet in a single layer.

5. Bake for 20-25 minutes until zucchini fries are golden and crispy.

6. Serve the baked Parmesan zucchini fries with your favorite dipping sauce.

Greek Yogurt Berry Parfait

Ingredients:

- 1 cup plain Greek yogurt

- 1 cup mixed berries (strawberries, blueberries, raspberries)

- 1 tablespoon honey or agave syrup (optional)

- 2 tablespoons chopped nuts (almonds, walnuts, or pistachios)

- Fresh mint leaves for garnish

Preparation:

1. In serving glasses or bowls, layer plain Greek yogurt with mixed berries.

2. Drizzle honey or agave syrup (if using) over the yogurt and berries.

3. Sprinkle chopped nuts on top.

4. Garnish with fresh mint leaves before serving.

Dark Chocolate-Dipped Strawberries

Ingredients:

- 1 cup dark chocolate chips or chopped dark chocolate (70% cocoa or higher)

- 12-15 fresh strawberries, rinsed and dried

Preparation:

1. Line a baking sheet with parchment paper.

2. In a microwave-safe bowl, melt the dark chocolate chips in 30-second intervals, stirring in between until smooth.

3. Dip each strawberry into the melted chocolate, coating about three-quarters of the berry.

4. Place dipped strawberries on the prepared baking sheet.

5. Refrigerate for 15-20 minutes until the chocolate is set.

Avocado Chocolate Mousse

Ingredients:

- 2 ripe avocados, peeled and pitted

- 1/4 cup unsweetened cocoa powder

- 1/4 cup honey or maple syrup

- 2 teaspoons vanilla extract

- Pinch of salt

- Fresh berries for garnish

Preparation:

1. In a food processor or blender, combine ripe avocados, cocoa powder, honey or maple syrup, vanilla extract, and a pinch of salt.

2. Blend until smooth and creamy, scraping down the sides as needed.

3. Transfer the avocado chocolate mousse to serving bowls or glasses.

4. Chill in the refrigerator for at least 30 minutes before serving.

5. Garnish with fresh berries before serving.

Chia Seed Pudding

Ingredients:

- 1/4 cup chia seeds

- 1 cup unsweetened almond milk or coconut milk

- 1 tablespoon honey or agave syrup

- 1/2 teaspoon vanilla extract

- Fresh fruit for topping (berries, sliced bananas)

Preparation:

1. In a bowl or jar, mix chia seeds, almond milk or coconut milk, honey or agave syrup, and vanilla extract.

2. Stir well to combine and ensure there are no clumps of chia seeds.

3. Refrigerate the mixture for at least 2-3 hours or overnight, stirring occasionally until it thickens into a pudding-like consistency.

4. Serve the chia seed pudding topped with fresh fruit.

Frozen Banana "Ice Cream"

Ingredients:

- 3 ripe bananas, peeled and sliced

- 2 tablespoons unsweetened cocoa powder or peanut butter (optional)

- 1/4 cup chopped nuts or shredded coconut (optional)

Preparation:

1. Place sliced bananas on a parchment-lined baking sheet and freeze until firm, about 2 hours or overnight.

2. Transfer frozen banana slices to a food processor.

3. Blend the frozen bananas until smooth and creamy, scraping down the sides as needed. Add cocoa powder or peanut butter if desired for flavor variation.

4. Fold in chopped nuts or shredded coconut for added texture if desired.

5. Serve immediately for a soft-serve consistency or freeze for 30 minutes for a firmer texture.

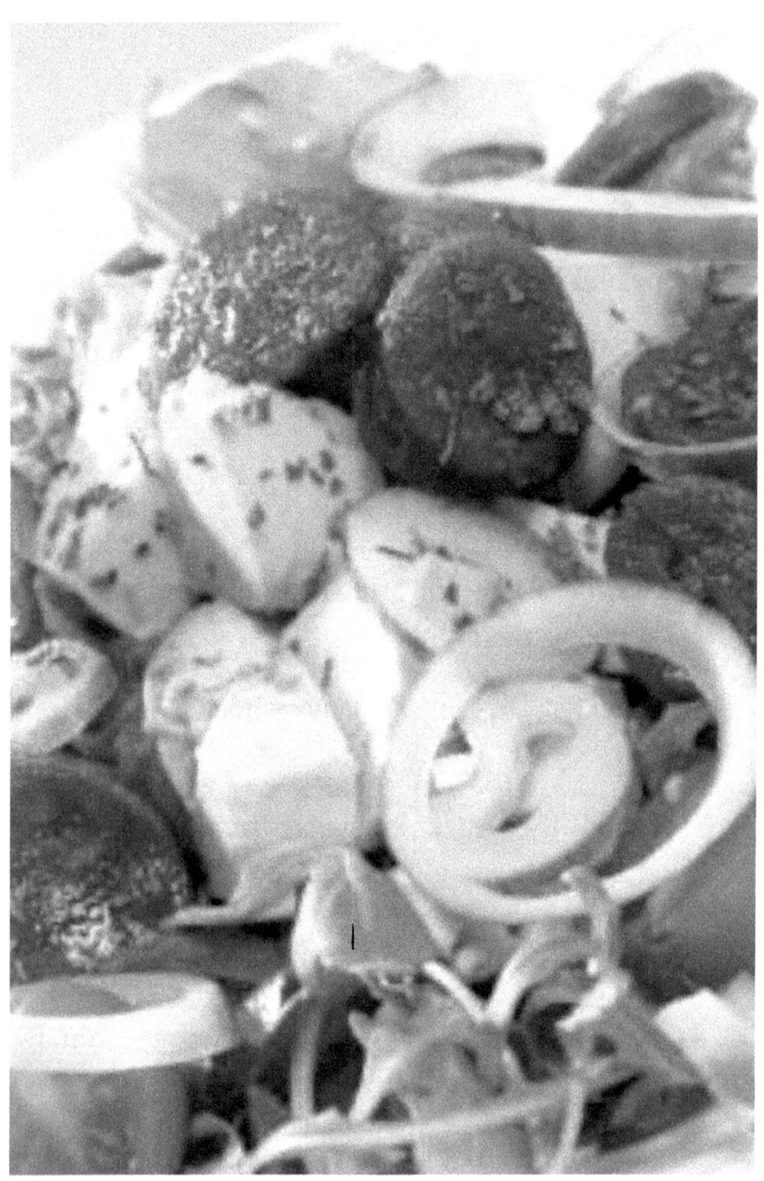

CHAPTER SEVEN

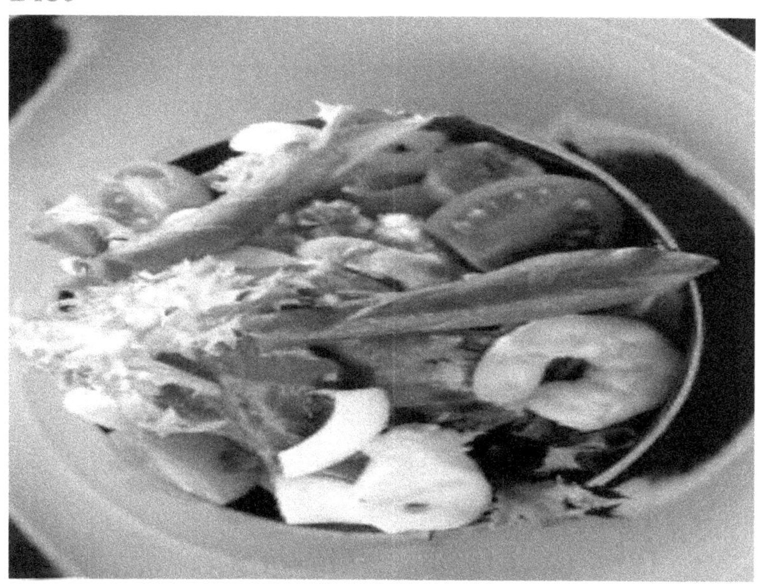

Grilled Vegetable Skewers

Ingredients:

- 1 zucchini, sliced

- 1 yellow squash, sliced

- 1 red bell pepper, diced

- 1 green bell pepper, diced

- 1 red onion, cut into chunks

- 8-10 cherry tomatoes

- 2 tablespoons olive oil

- 2 cloves garlic, minced

- 1 teaspoon dried herbs (such as thyme, rosemary, or oregano)

- Salt and pepper to taste

- Wooden skewers, soaked in water for 30 minutes

Preparation:

1. Preheat grill or grill pan over medium-high heat.

2. In a bowl, combine sliced zucchini, yellow squash, diced bell peppers, onion chunks, and cherry tomatoes.

3. In a small bowl, whisk together olive oil, minced garlic, dried herbs, salt, and pepper. Pour over the vegetable mixture and toss to coat evenly.

4. Thread the marinated vegetables onto the soaked wooden skewers.

5. Grill vegetable skewers for 8-10 minutes, turning occasionally, until vegetables are tender and slightly charred.

Sauteed Garlic Kale

Ingredients:

- 1 bunch kale, stems removed and chopped

- 2 tablespoons olive oil

- 3 cloves garlic, minced

- Juice of 1/2 lemon

- Red pepper flakes (optional)

- Salt and pepper to taste

Preparation:

1. Heat olive oil in a large skillet over medium heat.

2. Add minced garlic and red pepper flakes (if using). Cook for 1 minute until fragrant.

3. Add chopped kale to the skillet and sauté for 5-7 minutes until kale is wilted and tender.

4. Squeeze lemon juice over the sautéed kale and season with salt and pepper.

5. Stir to combine and serve as a nutritious side dish.

Ratatouille

Ingredients:

- 1 eggplant, diced

- 2 zucchinis, diced

- 1 red bell pepper, diced

- 1 yellow bell pepper, diced

- 1 onion, diced

- 2 cloves garlic, minced

- 2 cups diced tomatoes

- 2 tablespoons olive oil

- 1 teaspoon dried herbs (thyme, rosemary, or basil)

- Salt and pepper to taste

- Fresh basil leaves for garnish (optional)

Preparation:

1. Preheat oven to 375°F (190°C).

2. Heat olive oil in a large oven-safe skillet over medium heat. Add diced onion and minced garlic, sauté for 2-3 minutes until softened.

3. Add diced eggplant, zucchinis, bell peppers, diced tomatoes, dried herbs, salt, and pepper to the skillet. Stir to combine.

4. Transfer the skillet to the preheated oven and bake for 25-30 minutes until vegetables are tender.

5. Garnish with fresh basil leaves before serving this classic French dish.

Cauliflower Rice Stir-Fry

Ingredients:

- 1 head cauliflower, grated or processed into rice-like texture

- 2 tablespoons sesame oil

- 1 cup mixed vegetables (bell peppers, broccoli, carrots, etc.), chopped

- 2 tablespoons low-sodium soy sauce or tamari

- 2 cloves garlic, minced

- 1 teaspoon grated ginger

- Green onions for garnish (optional)

- Sesame seeds for garnish (optional)

Preparation:

1. In a large skillet or wok, heat sesame oil over medium-high heat.

2. Add minced garlic and grated ginger. Cook for 1 minute until fragrant.

3. Add chopped mixed vegetables and stir-fry for 3-4 minutes until slightly tender.

4. Add cauliflower rice to the skillet and stir-fry for another 3-4 minutes until cauliflower is cooked but not mushy.

5. Pour in low-sodium soy sauce or tamari. Stir well to combine.

6. Garnish with chopped green onions and sesame seeds before serving.

Roasted Root Vegetables

Ingredients:

- 2 carrots, peeled and cut into chunks

- 2 parsnips, peeled and cut into chunks

- 2 sweet potatoes, peeled and cut into chunks

- 2 tablespoons olive oil

- 1 teaspoon dried thyme

- 1 teaspoon paprika

- Salt and pepper to taste

- Chopped fresh parsley for garnish (optional)

Preparation:

1. Preheat oven to 400°F (200°C).

2. Place cut carrots, parsnips, and sweet potatoes on a baking sheet.

3. Drizzle with olive oil, sprinkle dried thyme, paprika, salt, and pepper. Toss to coat evenly.

4. Roast in the preheated oven for 25-30 minutes until vegetables are tender and caramelized.

5. Garnish with chopped fresh parsley before serving.

Berry and Spinach Salad

Ingredients:

- 4 cups baby spinach leaves

- 1 cup mixed berries (strawberries, blueberries, raspberries)

- 1/4 cup sliced almonds

- 2 tablespoons balsamic vinegar

- 1 tablespoon olive oil

- 1 teaspoon honey or agave syrup

- Salt and pepper to taste

Preparation:

1. In a large bowl, combine baby spinach leaves, mixed berries, and sliced almonds.

2. In a small bowl, whisk together balsamic vinegar, olive oil, honey or agave syrup, salt, and pepper.

3. Drizzle the dressing over the salad and toss to coat evenly.

Fruit Salad with Mint-Lime Dressing

Ingredients:

- 2 cups mixed fruits (pineapple, mango, kiwi, grapes, etc.), diced

- Juice of 2 limes

- 2 tablespoons honey or agave syrup

- 2 tablespoons chopped fresh mint leaves

Preparation:

1. In a bowl, combine diced mixed fruits.

2. In a small bowl, whisk together lime juice, honey or agave syrup, and chopped fresh mint leaves.

3. Drizzle the mint-lime dressing over the fruit salad and toss gently to combine.

Grilled Fruit Skewers

Ingredients:

- Assorted fruits (pineapple chunks, peach slices, strawberry halves, etc.)

- Wooden skewers, soaked in water for 30 minutes

- Honey or agave syrup for drizzling (optional)

- Ground cinnamon for sprinkling (optional)

Preparation:

1. Preheat grill or grill pan over medium heat.

2. Thread assorted fruits onto the soaked wooden skewers.

3. Grill fruit skewers for 3-4 minutes per side until grill marks appear and fruits are slightly caramelized.

4. Drizzle with honey or agave syrup and sprinkle with ground cinnamon if desired before serving.

Mango Salsa

Ingredients:

- 2 ripe mangoes, diced

- 1/2 red onion, finely chopped

- 1 jalapeño pepper, seeded and minced

- 1 red bell pepper, diced

- Juice of 1 lime

- 2 tablespoons chopped fresh cilantro

- Salt and pepper to taste

- Tortilla chips or cucumber slices for serving

Preparation:

1. In a bowl, combine diced mangoes, finely chopped red onion, minced jalapeño pepper, diced red bell pepper, lime juice, chopped fresh cilantro, salt, and pepper.

2. Stir to mix all ingredients well.

3. Serve mango salsa with tortilla chips or alongside cucumber slices.

Baked Cinnamon Apples

Ingredients:

- 4 apples (such as Granny Smith or Honeycrisp), cored and halved

- 2 tablespoons melted coconut oil or unsalted butter

- 2 tablespoons honey or maple syrup

- 1 teaspoon ground cinnamon

- Chopped nuts or granola for topping (optional)

- Greek yogurt for serving (optional)

Preparation:

1. Preheat oven to 375°F (190°C). Line a baking dish with parchment paper.

2. Place cored and halved apples in the baking dish, cut side up.

3. In a small bowl, mix melted coconut oil or butter, honey or maple syrup, and ground cinnamon.

4. Brush the mixture over each apple half.

5. Bake for 25-30 minutes until apples are tender and lightly golden.

6. Serve baked cinnamon apples warm, topped with chopped nuts or granola and a dollop of Greek yogurt if desired.

CHAPTER EIGHT

Brisk Walking or Power Walking:

- How to do it: Put on comfortable walking shoes. Start walking at a brisk pace, swinging your arms naturally. Maintain an upright posture and engage your core. Walk for at least 30 minutes per session, gradually increasing the duration or intensity as your fitness improves.

Running or Jogging:

- How to do it: Warm up by walking briskly, then transition into a light jog or run. Maintain proper form, landing softly on the balls of your feet and using your arms for momentum. Start with short distances or intervals, gradually increasing your pace or distance over time.

Cycling:

- How to do it: Hop on a bicycle and start pedaling. Whether it's outdoor cycling or using a stationary bike, maintain a steady pace. Adjust resistance or incline levels to challenge yourself. Aim for 20-30 minutes per session, gradually increasing the duration or intensity.

Squats:

- How to do it: Stand with feet shoulder-width apart. Lower your body as if sitting back into an imaginary chair, keeping your chest up and knees behind your toes. Push through your heels to return to the standing position. Aim for 3 sets of 10-15 reps.

Push-Ups:

- How to do it: Start in a plank position, hands slightly wider than shoulder-width apart. Lower your body until your chest nearly touches the floor, then push back up. Modify by doing knee push-ups if needed. Aim for 3 sets of 8-12 reps.

Plank:

- How to do it: Get into a push-up position but with forearms on the ground. Keep your body in a straight line from head to heels, engaging your core muscles. Hold for 30 seconds to 1 minute or longer as you progress.

Lunges:

- How to do it: Step forward with one leg and lower your body until both knees form a 90-degree angle. Keep your torso upright and step back to the starting position. Alternate legs. Aim for 3 sets of 10-12 reps on each leg.

Bicep Curls:

- How to do it: Hold a dumbbell in each hand with palms facing forward. Curl the weights toward your shoulders, keeping your elbows close to your body. Lower the weights back down. Aim for 3 sets of 8-12 reps.

Tricep Dips:

- How to do it: Sit on the edge of a sturdy chair or bench. Place your hands on the edge with fingers facing forward. Slide off the edge, supporting your body with your arms. Lower your body until your elbows are at 90 degrees, then push back up. Aim for 3 sets of 10-15 reps.

Swimming:

- How to do it: Swim laps in a pool or take part in water aerobics. Swimming engages various muscle groups while being gentle on the joints. Aim for 20-30 minutes of continuous swimming.

Jump Rope:

- How to do it: Use a jump rope and jump continuously at a moderate pace. This exercise is excellent for cardiovascular health. Start with intervals of 1-2 minutes and gradually increase the duration as your endurance improves.

High-Intensity Interval Training (HIIT):

- How to do it: Perform short bursts of intense exercises (like sprinting, jumping jacks, or burpees) followed by brief periods of rest or lower intensity activity. For example, sprint for 30 seconds, then walk for 1 minute. Repeat for several cycles.

Yoga:

- How to do it: Engage in yoga poses and sequences that focus on flexibility, balance, and relaxation. Poses like downward dog, warrior poses, and child's pose can improve flexibility. Follow guided yoga sessions or attend classes for proper guidance.

Pilates:

- How to do it: Pilates exercises emphasize core strength, stability, and flexibility. Moves like the hundred, leg circles, and bridges are commonly used. Attend classes or follow online tutorials to learn proper techniques.

Stretching:

- How to do it: Incorporate stretching exercises into your routine to improve flexibility and prevent muscle stiffness. Perform stretches for major muscle groups, holding each stretch for 15-30 seconds without bouncing.

Deadlifts:

- How to do it: Stand with feet shoulder-width apart, knees slightly bent. Bend at the hips and knees, lowering your torso while keeping your back straight. Grab a weighted barbell or dumbbells, stand back up by pushing through your heels. Aim for 3 sets of 8-10 reps.

Pull-Ups:

- How to do it: Use a pull-up bar. Grab the bar with an overhand grip, hands slightly wider than shoulder-width apart. Pull yourself up until your chin clears the bar, then lower yourself down. Modify using resistance bands or an assisted pull-up machine if needed. Aim for 3 sets of 5-8 reps.

Box Jumps:

- How to do it: Find a sturdy box or platform. Stand facing the box, bend your knees, and jump explosively onto the box. Land softly on the balls of your feet, then step back down. Start with a lower platform and gradually increase height as you progress. Aim for 3 sets of 8-10 jumps.

CONCLUSION

South Beach Diet Cookbook, serves as a testament to the harmony between health-conscious choices and culinary delight. It encapsulates more than just a collection of recipes; it's a comprehensive guide that embraces the essence of wholesome eating, proving that healthy food can be delicious, satisfying, and diverse.

Through this culinary compendium, individuals seeking to embark on a journey toward improved well-being will find a wealth of flavorful options. From vibrant salads bursting with fresh ingredients to comforting main courses and guilt-free desserts, each recipe embodies the fundamental principles of the South Beach Diet—promoting lean proteins, healthy fats, and low-glycemic index carbohydrates.

Beyond the kitchen, this cookbook is an invitation to adopt a lifestyle that celebrates mindful eating and nurtures a profound connection between nutrition and vitality. It empowers individuals to make informed choices, paving the way for sustained health improvements and a renewed sense of wellness.

As you turn the final pages of the "South Beach Diet Cookbook," let its culinary inspiration linger in your kitchen. Embrace the joy of cooking and savoring wholesome meals that not only nourish your body but also invigorate your spirit. Let this cookbook be a guiding light on your ongoing quest for a healthier, more vibrant life.

With its treasure trove of flavorful recipes and a holistic approach to healthy eating, the "South Beach Diet Cookbook" stands as a testament to the belief that achieving wellness doesn't mean sacrificing taste. It's a celebration of the extraordinary potential of food to nourish, energize, and delight—a culinary compass guiding you toward a more fulfilling and healthful existence.

www.ingramcontent.com/pod-product-compliance
Lightning Source LLC
Chambersburg PA
CBHW072132270726
48661CB00019BA/1664